Testimonials for:

RELEASE THOSE STUBBORN POUNDS

"This book is powerful and created deep exploration! It's a **vulnerable approach that's honest and real** and allows you to evaluate what health means in all facets of your life."

—Raushawna Price,
Author of *Be a Giver of Awesomeness*

"I loved Release Those Stubborn Pounds because it made me not just try a diet again, but to take the time to identify what is going on in my mind and in my body. It helped me **find ways I was sabotaging myself** and taught me ways to figure out why and what I could do to change."

—LM

"I have done every diet known to man, tried all the products, pills and recipes…and then I read this book! **No longer am I looking outside of myself to reach my goals and better my health.** Thank you so much Marjie for showing me how to work on not only my weight, but my whole being and outlook. This book is a must read for anyone wishing to lose weight, gain better health and most of all make your life your own!"

—Julie

"This book is **encouraging, motivating, empowering** and overall fantastic! I have struggled with losing weight and carrying around baggage over the years. Working through each session in this book allowed me to release stress which in return opened head space to truly focus on my weight issues. Marjie is a genuine, unique coach that encourages me to put my needs first."

—Amy

"Amazing book with **so much insight** on issues that I have faced in my journey for health. I can't wait to read more from this author!"

—Evelyn

"Loved this book! My favorite thing is that it deals with the **reasons behind the over-eating.** No preaching or "just do this." Marjie is very much in the trenches with us and guides through personal experience. This book **gently** aids in exploring the reasons we struggle to love ourselves and walks you into safe spaces to do that. Great imagery, stories and examples we can all relate to and understand. Very thought-provoking for every woman to consider her worth and be guided to a healthier version of herself. Highly recommend."

—Michelle D.

"I am thankful for the grace and the laying down of shame as I step forward wanting change. My vulnerability and willingness to begin were **met with gentleness and hope.**"

—M

"This book made me think of what is weighing my heart down. **It took away the "Why are you eating so much?" guilt** to look at my overall behavior."

—S. Lawrence

Release THOSE STUBBORN POUNDS

A gentle approach to lose what weighs you down

MARJIE METZ

Copyright © 2021 Marjie Metz

All rights reserved. No part of this book may be reproduced in any form without permission in writing from the author, except in the case for brief quotations, reviews, and articles.

Published 2021

Disclaimer: The information, ideas, and recommendations contained in this book are not intended as a substitute for medical advice or treatment. The client examples shared in this book are about real people and real events, but some details may have been changed or omitted for the privacy of those clients.

ISBN: 978-1-7362338-0-1

Cover and interior design: TeaBerryCreative.com

Editing: Natasa from The Author Incubator, Marnie Hammar, Michelle Diekmeyer, Debbie Hitchcock

Author's Photo Courtesy of: John Metz

To my family,

thank you for loving me, supporting me, and allowing me the time and space I needed to heal.

CONTENTS

Chapter 1	Introduction	1
Chapter 2	My Story	5
Chapter 3	The RELEASE Process	13
Chapter 4	Realize Your Potential	17
Chapter 5	Eat for Nourishment	25
Chapter 6	Listen to Your Body	33
Chapter 7	Evaluate Your Thoughts	39
Chapter 8	Adjust Your Responses	47
Chapter 9	Seek Understanding	55
Chapter 10	Enjoy Your Life	65
Chapter 11	You Are Worth It!	73
Chapter 12	What Do You Want?	79
	Acknowledgement	83
	About the Author	85

Chapter 1
INTRODUCTION

I remember checking out at the grocery store with my young kids and seeing a friend from high school. I was so embarrassed about how I looked that I pretended to not see her and quickly walked out the door. I missed an opportunity to connect with someone who had been very special to me…because of the way I thought I looked. Have you ever experienced that?

Have you ever looked in your closet for something to wear and thought, "I have nothing to wear!" Even though there are plenty of options…you just don't like how you look in any of them. And then you have to resort to your "fat" jeans again.

Have you ever been so consumed with counting calories and evaluating your food choices that deciding on a meal became a complicated affair? Have you made deals with yourself about having this or that food and then putting in extra effort at the gym to "work it off?"

Have you looked at skinny people thinking with envy how fortunate they are to be able to "eat whatever they want" while you just look at food and gain weight?

Have you worried about what example you are setting for your children?

Have you felt like you are observing your life more than actually living in it? You want to do more with your family, but feel like you can't. And the opposite—not wanting to do things with your family, even when you can. It's easier to shy away and hide than face the fear of putting yourself out there. Even with those closest to you.

Have you ever volunteered to take the picture, so you don't have to be in it?

I have felt and lived all of these scenarios.

I remember feeling so frustrated with my life, how I looked and not having the energy I wanted, and then lashing out at my kids in anger. It was ugly. That's when I knew I needed to get help. I could not keep hurting my kids out of frustration with myself. That was not being fair to them. They deserved better than that. I used that to propel me as I sought out answers and found the help I needed.

What's your story? How is excess weight holding you back? What opportunities might you be missing? Do you see yourself hurting others when you are upset with yourself?

You will not find judgment or condemnation in any of these pages. I've been there. I've walked the road. I've battled for my own sense of peace and to be the wife and mother that I wanted to be. I know it's hard. I'm so proud of you for picking up this book.

Are you willing to exercise your imagination with me for a moment? I want to paint a picture for you. I want you to imagine you are on a wonderful cruise. You bought that special dress that makes you feel amazing. You wear it to dinner and feel confident with how you look. You are proud of the work you have put in and the example you are to your family. You enjoy the wonderful meal, guilt-free...even dessert. You know how to balance nourishing your body with allowing yourself treats. You enjoy good relationships with your immediate family. You are able to be present in the moment, not stressing about your looks and what's happening next, just being in the moment. If you are single, you feel confident in who you are, with or without a significant other. If you have a family, because you are not hyper-focused on your own internal issues, you have the capacity to talk your children through a fight, with an even temper. Whatever the scenario, you have an amazing life and you know it.

That's what I want for you. Whether your picture of ideal lines up with the one I just painted or not, I want to help you live *your* definition of ideal. I am here to help you unlock your potential and help shift your body out of fat storage mode so you can *release what's weighing you down* and enjoy your amazing life!

Chapter 2
MY STORY

Over the years, I have had many meltdown moments that have forced me to face issues I tried to avoid. There were times when I took on too much or allowed too much stress in my life and was not the mom I wanted to be for my kids. There were times that I did not eat in ways that nourished my body and I suffered the consequences of those choices. I experienced rough emotional times because I let my mind get unhealthy and out of balance. These meltdown moments gave me an opportunity to stop, evaluate, and readjust how I had been living my life to allow for something new. I thank God that I have a kind and supportive husband who helped me through each dip (sometimes a nosedive) and helped me get back on my feet. I would not be who I am today without his love and support. Thanks Eric!

Although I could not see it then, I am truly grateful for all of these hard times. They caused me to have a breakthrough that I didn't even know I needed. Each of these breakthroughs made me grow and stretch in ways I could not have imagined.

Breakthrough #1:
I had my boys nineteen months apart and when they were four and two and a half, I had my daughter. The next year we moved to a new house. I think I ran on adrenaline for another year or so, and then I crashed. I just couldn't handle things. Everything felt overwhelming. I went on medication and noticed a difference within a week. I could handle more things, I felt better, the kids did not irritate me as much, and I could exercise again because I had energy. After many months of feeling stable, I slowly weaned off the medication.

WHAT I LEARNED: Prioritizing my mental health is just as important as my physical health.

Breakthrough #2:
A few years later I had our fourth child. The kids were so excited to have a baby brother! Then, he started crying...*a lot*...and I didn't know what to do to help him. Having three other children did not prepare me for this. He would cry like he was in pain and nothing seemed to help. We finally figured out five different things that contributed to his discomfort and then, miraculously right at four months, he stopped crying! I set him down in his bouncy seat... and he didn't cry! I remember looking around the room to see if anyone else noticed he was sitting there and content...no crying! During this same time, our oldest started having mild panic attacks when I would take him to school, stomach issues, and a few other things. We decided to homeschool him to try and alleviate some of his stress. Newborn...and homeschooling...and keeping up with the other two kids in school...a great idea, right? Actually, it wasn't as bad as I thought because my oldest was a huge help with the

baby. I could not have survived that time without him. And they are still close to this day.

Again, I was running on adrenaline, trying to get through each day and do what I needed to do for my kids. Those trying few months really took a toll on my health over the next year. I gained weight, was exhausted, and had a hard time dealing with everything. I just didn't feel like myself anymore. I kept hoping things would get better. They didn't. After (another) crying episode, Eric said, "It's time to call the doctor." I knew he was right, but I didn't want to go back on medication. I met with my doctor and told her how hard things were. She wanted to put me on medication, but I didn't really want to. She said, "Honey, I just want to help you be able to enjoy your life." I cried. Hard. That's exactly what I wanted to be able to do too. I chose to go on the medication. Not because I wanted to, but for my family. They deserved more. I did start to feel better on the medication, but that did not solve my weight and energy issues.

WHAT I LEARNED: My body has limits; lack of sleep and excess stress can cause damage.

Breakthrough #3:
A group of friends decided to train so that we could run the Disney Princess Half Marathon. Great! Here was the motivation to get me running and lose the weight. The only problem was, although it did help, it was not as much as I had hoped. After the longer runs, I would be hurting, exhausted, and pretty much out of commission. I still could not lose the "spare tire" I felt around my midsection. I thought, "This is the most I have worked out in years! I'm eating pretty well…what is the problem? Why can't I lose any more

weight?" I started doing research because I just didn't know why my body wouldn't release the extra weight. While researching, I learned about negative side effects of the medication I was on, I learned about functional medicine, and that there could be underlying issues affecting my health. After meeting with a functional medicine doctor, I learned I had a large yeast overgrowth (that caused weight gain, brain fog, irritability, low energy); low stomach acid (from too much stress) that impaired my digestion; and my body was under too much stress (circumstantial, emotional, and physical from over-exercising), all of which had taken a toll on my adrenal glands. Because my body had been under way too much stress, he recommended the following: only walking or yoga, targeted supplements, less processed foods and more fresh foods, eating a low glycemic diet, and making adjustments to decrease my stress. While implementing all of this, I worked out less, ate more, and lost weight. Inflammation was reduced in my body, so I lost the "puffy" look that I had. With killing off the yeast and eating low-glycemic foods, my energy came back, my brain cleared, and I felt strong and confident again.

WHAT I LEARNED: How to work with my body to release excess weight.

Breakthrough #4:
I remember coming home one night after shopping and being so wound up emotionally over a number of situations. I was so worked up that I couldn't even communicate with Eric. He wanted to know what was going on, but I asked him to just leave me alone because I was afraid I would unleash all of this pent-up emotion on him and be mean when it had nothing to do with him. He didn't understand,

but gave me space. A few days later I remember driving home from dropping off my son at a baseball game. I sensed that I was supposed to stop and take a picture of a building. I found a side road to pull over so that I could get a better view of the structure. It was an old shed. The shed was so unkempt that bushes had grown on the inside and were taking over. I sensed God whisper to me, "This is your mind right now. You have let so many lies, burdens, and worries take over." I started crying. I could totally see that! Yes, I had let so many things take over. I went home and started a journal entry listing out all the things I was worried and upset about and all the lies that I sensed I had allowed to take root and grow. It took a couple of weeks to unravel the mess in my head. As I did, I imagined myself uprooting the weeds and overgrown bushes and taking control of my mind. It was hard work, but what a beautiful thing it was to feel free and in control of my thoughts again.

WHAT I LEARNED: Sometimes I have to work for my mental peace.

Breakthrough #5:
A few years later, I had lost the excess weight, but I still felt "heavy." I had a lot of emotional pain that had been festering for years. I tried to push it back, but it just kept rising to the surface. I sought out counseling. I tried to make adjustments in some stressful relationships. I journaled. I prayed. Those things helped, but what really made a difference was when I learned the Listening and Inner Healing Prayer process of bringing my pain to God in prayer and asking him to speak into those areas. These prayer times brought deep healing and a sense of release that I felt spiritually, emotionally, mentally, and physically.

WHAT I LEARNED: God cares about my pain.

The last two breakthroughs were more gradual and happened over time. Rather than specific events that happened, they were shifts in how I viewed myself and my life. These shifts allowed me to experience more freedom and joy than I knew was possible.

Mindset Shift #1:

I grew up feeling like a victim of my circumstances. I could not control what was going on around me at that time and I was powerless to change the negative environment my parents created in our home. This mindset stayed with me even into adulthood and caused me to feel like a "prisoner" and "victim" in my own home—even as a *happily* married woman with children I *wanted*. This mindset caused a lot of fights and misunderstandings in our marriage. It also added a lot of emotional pain to neutral situations that I saw through the lens of me being the victim. After doing a lot of emotional and spiritual work, I realized that I *can* control my mindset about my own life. I *get to* decide what I want my life to look like. *I* am in charge of my decisions. Instead of keeping the victim mindset, I traded it in for being an active participant in my own life and creating a life I love.

WHAT I LEARNED: I have a choice.

Mindset Shift #2:

As I began to be an active participant in my own life and make decisions from a place of growth and freedom, I felt stronger and more empowered. Holding myself accountable to change; to grow; and take on new things was invigorating! I went through Health

Coach and Life Coach trainings. I took on coaching clients. I went through Revelation Wellness® to be a Group Fitness Instructor. I started teaching fitness classes that make women stronger from the inside out. Learning to make decisions based on what *I wanted* caused me to be happier and more content. I realized I did not have to wait for Eric to make me happy. Being content within myself was my responsibility, not his. My relationships with my children shifted as well. They were not "holding me hostage" in my life anymore. I could make decisions that I needed to make for *me*. I saw them through new eyes and could appreciate who they were because my needs were met. This enabled me to have more capacity to love and serve them. I could finally look at my life and see that I loved being in it!

WHAT I LEARNED: How to be content with *my* life.

Can you see this process? Each breakthrough and mindset shift brought more freedom—physically, mentally, emotionally, and spiritually. That's why I had to write this book. I just can't keep all of this goodness to myself. I *have* to share it with you! I don't know your story and I don't know what freedom looks like for you, but I challenge you to be open. Be open to not only lose physical weight, but see if there are other areas where you are "carrying weight" that may need to be released as well.

Chapter 3
THE RELEASE PROCESS

Are you ready for your breakthrough? Are you ready to learn how to work with your body to release the excess weight? Great! Keep reading…

I wrote this RELEASE process from my personal journey and from that of my clients. There are ways you can unknowingly tell your body to store fat. I want to uncover these for you so you can learn how to turn off that message and continue on your weight loss journey. I want you to work smarter, not harder. In this book, we will go through each step of the RELEASE process and see why those excess pounds are sticking around. There are so many diet plans and promises out there, how do you know which one is right for you? That's actually why I have a process that I will walk you through. Each body is unique and different in what works and what doesn't. As you learn to tune in to your body, you can determine what is the best way to nourish your body by identifying its specific needs.

Here is an overview of the process:

R—Realize Your Potential
E—Eat for Nourishment
L—Listen to Your Body
E—Evaluate Your Thoughts
A—Adjust Your Responses
S—Seek Understanding
E—Enjoy Your Life

This process is about learning to be aware of what's going on internally and dialing in to your thoughts and your body to see what messages they have for you. Your body is beautifully designed to protect you and it's been doing a fantastic job! I don't believe it's a coincidence that you picked up this book. Of all the weight loss books out there, you found mine. I trust you will find keys in the following pages to unlock hidden reasons why your body is stuck where it is. I'm so thankful you found me and that I get to be on this journey with you. I can't wait to see how you grow and shift and change.

I'm not sure how frustrating or hurtful your weight loss journey has been for you so far. For some of my clients, I know it has been very painful and a lot of hard work. Can you do me a favor? Can you tell yourself it's going to be okay? Things are going to get better. You *will* find an answer. You *will* learn how to work with your body. Can you believe that? Can you please open up space in your heart for a good experience to come through these pages? Maybe you will even enjoy the process! When I'm working with clients, we frame the journey as discovering, learning, and finding new opportunities. Maybe you have spent some time in the guilty, shaming, self-loathing camp. Can I invite you into a new camp? The "I believe I can change and create a new experience for myself" camp. It's a fun place to be and it's where you belong.

If you feel as if you have tried everything and are wanting to finally lose the excess weight and have a different experience, you have to *do* something different. That is what will make the difference between wanting to change and actually changing. Are you ready for that? Because you are reading this book, my guess is that you ARE ready—you are ready to create something new. To represent that, I want you to purchase a very special notebook. One that makes you happy to look at and that can represent the beautiful changes you are about to make. As you go through this book, see the questions and *Take Action* sections as invitations into creating change for yourself. Take time to process the questions, journal, and be thoughtful about your answers. Work through this book at your own pace. Some people will read through it all, then go back and work through the questions. Others might take their time and work through the questions slowly and sit in a chapter for a while before moving forward. The pace that works for you is the "right" way for going through this book. As you work through these chapters, imagine I am sitting in a comfy chair right across from you sharing my experience, coaching you through the following process, asking questions, and cheering you on as you unlock your potential.

Chapter 4
REALIZE YOUR POTENTIAL

Do you remember dreaming and pretending when you were little? You had the joy and freedom to dream and imagine whatever you wanted. No one told you to dream or pretend, you just did. That is one of the joys of being a child. Somewhere along the line, we have cut off that part of ourselves for various reasons. I would like to ask you to resurrect that part of your brain. Are you willing to try and do that for the following mental exercise? Part of my job as a coach is to grow and stretch what you see as possible for yourself. I don't know exactly why your body is stuck where it is right now, but I do know that in order for change to happen, I have to help motivate your brain to a space where it can accept that change. There's a common saying, "Where the brain goes, the body follows." This chapter is all about allowing the brain to open up to new possibilities so that your body can begin acting on a new reality. Are you ready?

Let's say that you are Cinderella standing in the garden, wanting to go to the ball (or fill in your wish here), but you feel like you can't. I, your lovely fairy godmother, appear. I can grant your wish, but it must be something that matters very deeply to you. What do you want for yourself? What would matter more than anything else if you could change it? Part of your wish can involve losing weight, but there has to be a deeper desire as well. Describe in detail what that would be. What does it feel like? What will it look like? What is different about you?

> *Take Action:* Remember how I mentioned in the last chapter about "wanting" to change versus *actually* changing, and that you have to *do* something different? Now is the time to make the choice and *act* on that! Use the special notebook you purchased and write down your wish with as much detail as you can. Tell yourself this is a safe place for you to express yourself. Take time to really sit in this and let the words flow as you give a voice to your dream. When you finish, I would like you to summarize the main points of your wish for yourself. When I work with my coaching clients, I challenge them to write their statements in present tense, with positive wording and in a compelling way. To help you understand, I will share my wish: *I am comfortable in my own skin. I am fit and strong. I have healthy relationships with my family. I wake up each day looking forward to what is on my calendar.*

Now it's your turn. Consider these statements to help bring your wish to life: *I look like…I see myself trying to…The traits I embody are…What's different about me is that I…Others would notice that I…I am happy that I…*

How does it feel to see that in writing? Exciting? Terrifying? Comforting? Somewhere in between? Hopefully, it will invoke a strong emotion…that's when you know you have landed on the right thing. Good job for allowing yourself to dream and express what is really inside you. Nice work!

Let's keep going...

Imagine for a moment that your wish has come true. Close your eyes and imagine this new version of you. Can you see her? Can you feel how different she is? What is she hearing, seeing, feeling? Describe how she is different than the current version of you. What possibilities open up for her, that were not possible for you before? What is she doing that you could not do? If you have a clear picture, ask her what advice she has for the current version of you.

Write down what you observed and if you heard anything. Now that you have a clear picture of what it is you want and what it would feel like to be that future version of yourself, are you getting a sense of what might need to change for you? Anything you need to do differently? What becomes more important? What becomes less important?

> ***Take Action:*** Take a moment now and just sit in all that we have discussed so far. Read back over your answers. *Don't miss this step.* It may seem insignificant, but it's absolutely vital! This gives your mind permission to believe that things *can* be different for you; that it's *possible* for you to have a different experience. Allow these images to expand your brain and the potential they hold for you. As you do this, new opportunities will open up for you in your thoughts that did not seem to exist before. Your brain was not trained (yet) to see these opportunities as possibilities for you, so it discounted them. Now that you are drawing a picture of who it is you really want to be, your brain will now be looking for ways to carry out this new reality.

This new reality happened with a client who came to me for weight loss. We were going over the same questions that I just had you work through to uncover what she really wanted out of our time together. Besides losing weight, she wanted to start enjoying cooking healthy food for her family. She even laughed as she said it because it seemed a bit of a stretch for her. We wrote out, "I am fifteen pounds lighter and I enjoy cooking creatively for my family." And guess what...At the end of our time working together, she had lost the weight *and* somewhere along the line she had actually started *enjoying* cooking delicious, healthy meals for her family! She had given her brain a direction to go, so her brain found ways to actually make it happen.

In order to help you succeed as you start on this journey toward the new and improved you, we need to go over some key ingredients of success. I would be setting you up for failure if I didn't mention these. How many times have you started (another) new diet plan, you're all ramped up to get started and you say, "*This* time will be different! I will stay on track with my exercise routine and the pounds will just melt off. Nothing can stop me!" And after one week...you wonder what in the world happened to all that excitement and determination.

There are three things we need to determine for lasting change:

1. What is your *internal* motivation?
2. What is your anchor?
3. What are you willing to give up?

WHAT IS YOUR INTERNAL MOTIVATION?

This is why it is so important to identify what it is you *truly* want; it can't just be a "I want to lose twenty pounds one day" kind of thing. It must matter *deeply* to you. If you don't accomplish this goal, it will crush you. Maybe ask yourself, "*Why* do I want to lose these twenty pounds? Why does it matter whether I lose them or not? How will my life be better if I lose them? Why is it a negative thing to stay where I am?" Dig down a bit and get to the root of *why* it matters to lose weight. If it's just to lose weight, that's an *external* motivation and as soon as you are uncomfortable or feeling self-conscious or you don't feel like working out…"wanting to lose twenty pounds" just doesn't matter as much as your comfort in that moment! You must dig deeper into your *internal* motivation to get over your discomfort in the moment to push through and work toward your goal.[1]

For me, it was my family. I was overweight, felt puffy, was irritable and self-conscious, had low energy, and felt anxious and depressed. I just couldn't function the way I wanted to for myself or my family. I didn't like who I was as a wife. As a mom, I didn't like how I was treating my children. I decided there had to be a better way. I chose to get on medication, change how I was eating, get moving and learn how to take care of myself, to take better care of my family. It wasn't just about looking better. It was deciding *who* I wanted to be for my family. Did I want my children to remember me as being depressed, angry, and tired all the time? *No!* I decided we had had enough of that mom. I decided I wanted *more* for myself and my family. So, I had to pour my effort and energy into creating that for them.

---

[1] I picked up the concept of internal motivation from Shad Helmstetter, "Self-Talk and Motivation," in *What to Say When You Talk to Yourself: Powerful New Techniques to Program Your Potential for Success* (New York: Gallery Books, 2017).

Take Action: Can you see the difference? The gravity of that situation prompted me to keep moving forward, even when it became difficult. What's your story? Why do you want to lose weight? What circumstances are becoming too painful for you to stay the same? Write out your story and then imagine you are sharing it with me.

WHAT IS YOUR ANCHOR?

Let's go back to the future version of yourself for a moment. Can you see her? How can you capture this? Is there a statement, a picture, a word...something that can remind you of her? In the coaching world, we call this an anchor.[2] It anchors you into that new, improved version of you. It's similar to a vision board—you post quotes and pictures and words that are meaningful and that you want to achieve. This step is important because in order to create something new, you *must* have a vision for where you are headed. If not, how will you know where you are going or when you have arrived?

An anchor serves two purposes. One, it reminds you of your vision and where you are headed so you stay on track. Two, it pulls you out of your current circumstance and connects you to your vision. This is especially important when you are tempted to eat a food you have committed to not having. Or your anchor gets you up off the couch and out for a walk, run, or to the gym. It helps you overcome the comfort of the moment and connect back to your

---

[2] I learned the concept of an anchor during my training to be a Health and Life Coach. I am sure many other concepts in this book are from that training, but it's hard to pinpoint them because they have just become a part of how I think and how I coach. This note is to give credit for my training. "Become a Health Coach" and "Life Coach" certifications through Health Coach Institute, August, 2015.

motivation for change. The anchor must be powerful enough to keep you grounded in the journey and meaningful enough to keep you inspired and moving forward.

Take Action: What is your anchor? What can remind you of the vision you are holding for yourself? A picture, a word, a phrase, a song? Where can you post your anchor so you see it every day?

WHAT ARE YOU WILLING TO GIVE UP?

You must consider this question if you want lasting changes. For me, I had to give up some of the foods I wanted to eat and some sedentary reading and entertainment time, but more than that…I had to give up on doubting myself, feeling insecure, and allowing anger and frustration to rule me. I could have easily stayed in the victim mode and said, "I have four kids and they are the reason I can't take care of myself and why I look this way." But I chose to do something about it. I didn't let my insecurity rule me and hide behind the weight and my kids.

I also gave up blaming. I decided my body and my life were *my* responsibility. I decided I wanted a better experience for my life…for my husband's sake, for my children's sake, for the future version of me that would want to be different. No matter what I'd experienced, I could create a new identity. And so can you!

Take Action: What about you? What are you willing to give up? If you knew it would be worth it, what would you be willing to surrender? What would the future version of you tell you? What will the trade-off be for giving this up?

If you worked through the questions and have a clear vision of what you want for yourself, great job! Can you feel this clarity? Can you see how getting in touch with your internal motivation, having an anchor, and giving up what's getting in your way…can you see the difference they will make? Do you feel yourself getting motivated and feeling empowered to make changes? I sure hope so. My friend, dare to dream. Change *is* possible and it's possible *for you*. You are worthy of so much more! You deserve it. Your family and friends deserve it. And the future version of you can't wait for you to step into what is possible for you!

If you are still unclear, that's totally fine! You can just pause and sit in this chapter for a bit and allow time for your vision to become clear. You are worth the time and effort to do this. Another strategy is to read through the rest of this book, answer the questions, and notice any clues you might receive about what it is you want for yourself. Keep a page in your notebook for gathering these clues and build your vision as you read. Don't worry about doing this the "right" way…whatever works for *you* is the right way of doing this. Take a deep breath, allow your brain and your body to relax. Tell yourself you are going on an adventure to discover what it is you want. Allow this to be a process of understanding *you*…what makes you tick, what works for your body, what makes you happy, what you want, what you don't want. I can't wait to see what you uncover!

Chapter 5
EAT FOR NOURISHMENT

Do you like being told what to eat? Are you like, "Just tell me the plan and I'll follow it"? Or, are you a "I like to create my own plan" kind of person? I will satisfy both needs in this chapter, but probably not in the way you might think. I don't have a specific eating plan spelled out for you in this program. I can hear some of you groan! I know, I know…hang in there with me!

I am confident there *is* a specific plan that will work for you, but finding that is where the fun begins! Your body is great at discerning what is beneficial for you and what is not. We have just ignored its signals and tried to follow the latest Facebook or Instagram trend. My goal is to help you learn to tune in to your body to determine what way of eating makes you function the best. I want to give you a list of foods that energize and empower you throughout your day and to know the foods that deplete your energy and zap your strength. How does that sound? Would you like to know what they are?

The tricky part is that it's not one-size-fits-all. What works for me, might not work for you and what works for you might not work for your best friend. The key is tuning into *your* body and learning what helps it and what hurts it. Most of us are not used to listening to our bodies, so it's like learning a new language. Are you up for this challenge?

Through my personal health journey, as well as helping my clients, I have learned the following questions to be the most helpful:

- How can I upgrade this?
- How did my body respond to that?
- What do I need right now?

HOW CAN I UPGRADE THIS?

Our food choices should nourish our bodies and give them what they need to function well. Just like if you filled a car with olive oil and expected it to run…it would not…and other people would look at you like you were crazy! Then, why do we eat fuel that is not designed to help our bodies and then get mad when they don't look or function like we want them to? So, the first step in eating for nourishment, is asking: How can I upgrade this?

An easy way to upgrade your food is to cook at home whenever possible. You don't always know what is going into food that you let others prepare for you; how long it's been sitting there; and if it's all natural or not. At home, you know what's going in your food and you get to choose the quality of that food. That's an upgrade. The easiest way to implement this upgrade is to maximize your time in the kitchen. Let's say you are grilling chicken for dinner. Grill two or even three times the amount you need for that dinner. Now you have a quick and easy protein source for other meals. Let's say you are making steamed broccoli as the side dish. Steam two or even three times the amount you need for that dinner. The broccoli can be added to a salad, stir-fry, soup, or a baked potato. You have just made it easy to upgrade your meals!

Another way to upgrade is to eat as many all-natural, organic foods that you can. The less chemicals and additives you eat, the better. According to Mike Mutzel, these chemicals have the potential to alter metabolic pathways, promote fat storage and disease.[3] That is exactly what we are trying to avoid! If you're interested in learning more about the science behind this, you can check out his book, *Belly Fat Effect*. For my kids, I really noticed a difference in their behavior when they ate certain commercially prepared treats with artificial coloring in them. For my one son, he became aggressive and would act out more, especially after having food or dinks that contained artificial red food coloring. I learned to check the treats and drinks at parties and gatherings. I tried to either bring something he could have or let him know I would make him something else at home. I had to be more intentional and proactive, but it made such a difference in his behavior that it was worth it!

Let's say for lunch you want to eat a turkey sandwich. How can you upgrade this? Is the turkey all natural with no preservatives? Do you have any veggies you can chop up to serve on the side? Do you have lettuce to make a lettuce wrap instead of using bread? Those are great ways to upgrade!

What about making macaroni and cheese for you kids (all natural, of course), how can you add value? You could add protein by serving it with a turkey roll-up (all-natural, preservative-free) or leftover chicken. You could add carrot and cucumber sticks and then finish it off with fruit. I learned this when the kids were little

---

3   Mike Mutzel, *Belly Fat Effect: The Real Secret About How Your Diet, Intestinal Health, and Gut Bacteria Help You Burn Fat* (Oregon: Wilsonville Media, 2014), 84.

and they would be hungry thirty minutes after lunch...how frustrating! By upgrading their lunch and adding in protein and fiber, they were satisfied longer. One of my kids' favorites was Chili Mac 'n Cheese—they still ask for it![4] I used brown rice pasta, beans, chili seasoning, chopped onions, butter and shredded cheddar. Can you see the upgrades? I added protein, fat and fiber; I made it more natural by using my own seasoning, and because I made it at home, I knew what ingredients were used. These are simple swaps or additions, but they can really increase the nutritional value of the meal.

To upgrade my daily choices, there are three things I have found to be the most beneficial: increasing my water intake, adding fiber and/or protein to each meal or snack, and eating more vegetables. [5]When I incorporate these three things my mind is clearer; I make better choices; I am more productive; I have a more positive outlook on my day; I have more patience for those around me; I have the energy I need to work out.

> *Take Action:* Think through your meals over the next few days. How can you upgrade them? Start reading labels for the foods you regularly purchase. How can you make them more natural and have less additives? Rather than fast food for a quick lunch at work, what if you packed leftovers from last night's dinner? What vegetables can you prepare to have on hand for easy side dish options? How can you incorporate drinking more water in your daily routine? Don't over-complicate this...I am not

---

[4] This recipe and more available at www.marjiemetz.com/release-resources
[5] For my favorite green drink recipe, check out www.marjiemetz.com/release-resources

asking you to revamp everything you eat! Just start making simple upgrades to the snacks and meals that you are already used to having.

HOW DID MY BODY RESPOND TO THAT?

The next question to consider is, "How did my body respond to that?" The more tuned in you can be to how your body responds to certain foods, the better able you will be to create a food list that uniquely works with your body. Just because it's good for someone else, doesn't mean it's right for your body. You can begin to decipher foods that your body is sensitive to as well as foods that your body says, "Yes! More please!" With my clients I have them record foods that energize them and foods that cause them to feel depleted and low in energy.

Consider this—if you have a personal trainer and they are telling you to replenish after your workout with a whey-based protein powder and you feel super heavy and then constipated later that night…is it really a healthy option for you? Maybe you can try a plant-based protein powder and see how your body responds to that. This is what is so vital about tuning in to your body…just because someone says it's healthy, doesn't mean it will work for *your* body.

One of my clients went through a cleanse with me and after removing certain foods, her sinuses cleared up after months of infections. Her body was trying to tell her there was a problem. Once she removed the problematic foods, her body could calm down and function normally again. Another client removed dairy from her diet and her headaches went away. She didn't even realize she had headaches that often, they had just become normal for her.

Take Action: Are you aware of how certain foods affect you? When you eat (add specific food), you feel light, energized, and clear-headed. When you eat (add specific food), you feel heavy, sluggish, and foggy. If you are not aware of how foods affect you, now is the perfect time to start tracking. You can create a simple food log in a notebook. Each day, write down the time you eat, what you eat, and what you drink. On the right side of the page, record any symptoms that you observe (headache, foggy brain, low energy, irritable, upset stomach, etc.). Keep your food log for at least seven days. This gives you an opportunity to look over your food choices and see if you can make any connections with certain foods and symptoms that you experience.[6]

WHAT DO I NEED RIGHT NOW?

This is the key question to ask if you struggle with emotional eating. So many times, out of habit, we go to food to solve a problem it was never designed to solve. We have been programmed to view food as so much more than fuel due to advertising and habits we have been taught. Media has hijacked these messages and sold us everything from fast food, to candy, to alcohol—and sold the message that it will buy happiness and joy and a sense of belonging. Has it delivered that for you? I know it hasn't for me! I want to divorce food from those marketing messages and reclaim food for what it is designed to be—nourishment.

What if you ate foods that nourished your body; only ate food when you were truly hungry; could stop eating when you were

---

[6] For a downloadable Food and Mood Log, go to www.marjiemetz.com/release-resources

satisfied; and allowed yourself to indulge in what you crave? Imagine what that could do for your body. Can you feel the freedom in eating that way? No calorie counting, no stressing over a perfectly balanced plate, no guilt. What a glorious day that would be! We would be functioning exactly as our creator designed us to function.

But, due to advertising and the messages we have been hearing for far too long, we associate feelings with food. Sad? Make brownies. Frustrated? Have a glass of wine. Missing a loved one? Eat a carton of ice cream. Crappy day at work? You deserve a special drink!

What if you could pause, identify what you are feeling and then ask the even deeper question: What do I need right now? That is when you have hit the jackpot! You cannot solve a problem you don't know. Here's the magic formula: **identify the feeling + identify the need = solve the real problem.**

When I was finally able to start using food for its original purpose, I felt a new level of freedom. Rather than feeling chained to food, craving it all the time, and then beating myself up for overdoing it, I now have a healthier relationship with food. I don't look to food to solve problems that it can't solve. I am better at identifying my feelings, my needs, and then I find ways to address them. That opens up the freedom to indulge in a craving when I have one. For example, I'm being totally honest here, once a month, you will find me making a pan of brownies…guilt-free brownies at that! Because I do not give in to cravings all the time, when I have a true craving for warm, gooey brownies when I am feeling super crummy, then I allow myself to enjoy them. That is the freedom that comes when you are able to name your feelings, your needs, and meet them.

Take Action: Do not judge or condemn yourself as you consider the following questions! Be in observation mode and do not make judgments about whether you are "good" or "bad" based on your answers. Your job is to *observe your behavior*. What motivates you to eat? Do you feel hungry? Do you eat to solve a problem? Do you eat to stuff your emotions? Do you eat out of boredom? Do you eat when you are stressed? Remember, no judgment! You are just observing your behavior. I'm trying to help you uncover areas where you have been turning to food and may not even realize it. Are you aware of what problems or emotions trigger you to turn to food? If not, when you notice yourself eating (and you know it's not true hunger), start asking yourself:

- What happened right before I started eating?
- What am I feeling right now?
- What do I need right now?
- How can I solve the real need that I have?

I know this might be a lot of information to take in. If you need to pause and sit in this chapter for a while, go ahead! Read back over the *Take Action* sections and take your time answering the questions. This chapter alone can cause major shifts in your health by changing your relationship to food. As you learn to upgrade your food choices, tune in and determine what is right for your body, and uncover your true needs—you are learning how to truly *nourish your body*. As you do this, and make the proper adjustments, your body will say, "Thank you! I have been waiting for you to hear me. Now I can release this excess weight and create more energy for you!" How does that sound?!

Chapter 6
LISTEN TO YOUR BODY

There are many factors that can contribute to turning on the fat storage message in your body. I want to highlight three areas that have made the most difference for me and my clients. To know if you need to make changes in these three areas, you need to learn how to listen to your body and see what it is trying to tell you.

HOW SLEEP HELPS WITH WEIGHT LOSS
Your body requires a certain amount of sleep to function optimally. That amount can be different for each one of us, but general recommendations are between seven to nine hours for adults, more for children. Why does that matter? While you are sleeping, your body is able to rest, repair, and do restorative work. If you consistently do not get enough sleep, your body cannot do the repair work that it needs to do and it will affect your waistline.[7] A lack of deep sleep is what caused me to gain weight and slip into a depression after I

---

7 Mike Mutzel, *Belly Fat Effect*, 129.

had my fourth child. As I shared earlier, he had such a rough time as an infant and it seemed like he did not stop crying for the first four months. Nothing I did could console him. That time really took a toll on my health. It took me years to finally feel like I had recouped from that trying time.

Not only does sleep help the body heal, but it also facilitates balanced hormones as well as more stable energy and moods. I'm sure you have felt the impact of these. Imagine a day when you did not get a full night's sleep and you did not have very much energy. What did you do? Most of us reach for high sugar, high caffeine options to try and get a shot of artificial energy. This overloads the body and puts it into a state of stress, which turns on the fat storage mode. The same thing can happen with a depressed or low mood. How do you respond? What do you reach for? You might reach for a quick mood lifter—sugar or caffeine. Again, putting the body into a state of stress which will turn on the fat storage mode.

My husband and I have said that getting enough sleep should be considered a spiritual discipline! That has made all the difference for all aspects of our health.

> **Take Action:** Do you sleep enough each night? How much sleep do you need to feel at your best? If you don't know, what can you do to try and figure that out? If you know you need more sleep, how can you start making that happen? What needs to change?

If you are a mom with a baby or young child, you may be laughing (or crying) reading over this section. You are in a totally different season! Your job is to recognize how important sleep is and to make it a priority. Go to bed early when you can; rest when you can;

nap whenever you get the chance; ask for and accept help whenever you can. *Do not* stay up late to finish chores—your health is more important than being caught up on chores! Trust me, prioritizing sleep not only helps your body but also helps you function better and allows you to be the mom you want to be during this season. What your house looks like is not as important as your health!

HOW YOU EAT CAN ENCOURAGE FAT STORAGE

Have you ever been in a rush and quickly ate your meal—then you either ate too much *or* you were hungry within the hour? This is a clue from your body; it is not just about the actual food you eat. The manner in which you consume your food also matters.

Another example is if you are really stressed about something and you eat a meal, then you end up with a stomachache afterward. Again, it's not just about what you are eating, but the state you are in when consuming your food. Eating in a state of stress forces the body to make a choice—to be prepared for the danger you are telling it is coming, *or* focus on digestion. Your brain will choose survival every time! That means it will divert the energy away from digestion and toward getting ready to survive the crisis. This means (you may have guessed it) your body must turn on fat storage mode to conserve energy and be ready to react quickly if needed. Slowing down metabolism is another way your body will try to help you through a perceived crisis.

The best thing you can do to solve this problem is to slow down, take a few breaths, and calm your body and your mind before enjoying your meal. This allows your body to focus on digestion and better utilize the nutrients in your food. This is a great reason to pause and thank God for your food, your family, whatever else comes to mind. A heart and mind focused on gratitude is a wonderful way to keep stress at bay! But I'm getting ahead of myself, more on that in the next chapter.

Take Action: Consider what state you are in when you eat. Are you calm? Stressed? Are you usually rushing? Or, relaxed and taking your time? How can you change things to allow for you to eat in a more relaxed state?

WHAT FORM OF MOVEMENT IS BEST FOR WEIGHT LOSS?
I prefer to use "movement" and "working out" instead of "exercise" because many people have negative associations with the word exercise. The correct answer to that question is—whatever type of movement you actually enjoy! If you hate running, don't torture yourself! Find some other form of movement that you actually enjoy. Do you like dancing? Find a dance-aerobic type class. Do you like gardening? Have a go at it! Do you like walking? Awesome! Do you like weight training? Then, go for it. The best form of exercise for weight loss is any type of movement that you enjoy and will do consistently. If you enjoy it, you will be more likely to stick with it longer and find it easier to fit in your schedule regularly. Don't make it more difficult than it has to be. I would rather you get in three to five sessions of something you enjoy each week, than trying to coerce and will yourself into going to the gym every day... and then not showing up. Not only are you not exercising, but you are mentally beating yourself up over it. How is that healthy?

Next, you need to consider: Does this give me energy or deplete me? After you do a workout (whatever you have chosen to do), notice how it impacts your body. Do you have more energy? Or, do you feel exhausted? This is your body giving you a clue. We tend to think, "If I just work out harder or longer, then I will lose more weight." That is not true. The season in my life when I was working out longer than I ever had, my body would not release the extra, stubborn pounds. I had put my body in such a state of stress that working out more was not helping. I had a functional medicine doctor tell me to stop working out so much. He prescribed walking and yoga and that was it. I ended up eating more (of the right foods for my body), working out less and not as hard, and my body began shedding pounds! So, don't miss this. Pay attention to the clues your body is giving you.

The activities that you choose to do for movement should energize you, lift your mood, and increase your self-confidence. If they exhaust you or cause you to feel worse about yourself, then give them up! They are not right for you. Tune into *your* body and see what messages it has for you about what type of movement is right for *you*.

Many clients ask, "How do I fit in movement in my already busy schedule?" I don't think that is the right question. The better question is, "What do I want for myself?" Look back at your description of your dream for yourself. If it has anything to do with less stress, less depression and anxiety, better moods, losing weight, feeling stronger, more confidence, better relationships… then movement is a necessary step to accomplishing those. The more you train and take care of your body, the more capacity you have in so many areas. What helps is shifting your mindset about exercise. Instead of it being a *have to*, let's change it into finding enjoyable ways to move and then it becomes a *get to*! For me, I have found that strength training two times per week and then short cardio sessions two to three times per week are what I enjoy. My cardio is running in my neighborhood or hopping on my stationary bike. Twenty to thirty minutes is all I need to burn off any excess stress, pray, and enjoy the process of getting stronger and fitter. Seeing results in my body and having more peace of mind are the outcomes that I receive and that keeps me motivated to show up the next day. If my focus is just on, "I have to work out five times this week," I would only workout once or twice, if that! If you connect deeply to the outcome of what you really want, then your workouts become the steps to help you get there.

Another way to think about it is if your tooth is hurting, would you cancel your appointment with the dentist? No, you wouldn't. If you are sick, would you cancel your appointment with the doctor? No, you would do whatever you need to do and get there. What if you could start seeing your whole health (mental, emotional, physical, and spiritual) the same way? Working out affects all of these areas and will improve your quality of life. What if you could start seeing your body as "sick" and movement is what you need to do to make it better? You make an appointment—a class, an online video, strengthening, etc.—and you keep it, knowing your very health depends on it.

> ***Take Action:*** What form of movement do you enjoy? What energizes you? What makes you feel exhausted? Is there something new you would like to try this week? Where can you add in thirty-minute time slots for movement?[8]

---

8   If you would like to try a class with me, check out www.marjiemetz.com/release-resources

Chapter 7
EVALUATE YOUR THOUGHTS

This chapter is so important! It may seem insignificant, but it can have a major impact on your progress toward your weight loss goal. You might be thinking, "What do my thoughts have to do with my weight loss? Is there really any connection?" I'm glad you asked, I am happy to explain the connection.

In the previous chapter I shared about when the body is in a state of stress, it can trigger the fat storage mode. Here's the thing, the body does not discern whether it is *perceived* stress or real stress. Imagine you step out in the road and you have to quickly jump back to avoid the car you didn't see—the body is thrown into a state of stress. Rightly so. That caused you to react quickly and the body had adrenaline and cortisol pumping to get you to act quickly. What you may not realize is that you can cause that same reaction in your body by what you are communicating with your mind. "I'm so late, I have to hurry!" "How will I get all of this finished?" "I don't even know what to have for dinner." "Should I accept this role or wait for something different?" These worries and concerns are running through your mind as you rush through your day. Can you feel the stress and tension? That is exactly how you can put yourself in a state of stress with your thoughts. And guess what that means—the body is slowing down metabolism and turning on fat storage to protect you and help you be ready for whatever is going to happen. In an emergency situation, you would say, "Thank you, body, for doing your job!" However, in dealing with everyday stressors, you can be turning on that same message and then be mad at your body for carrying out its job!

Mike Mutzel explains this very well in his book *Belly Fat Effect*, "For example, feelings such as loss of control, defeat, and work-related stress activate the stress response and are associated with obesity and diabetes. When this primitive survival response is over-stimulated, we suffer from poor sleep, reduced energy, depression, low motivation, reduced libido, high blood pressure, plaque buildup in blood vessels, stagnant digestion, immune system changes, inflammation, and increased levels of leptin and free radicals, all of which promote fat around the abdomen and adverse metabolic changes."[9]

Don't miss this part: "...feelings such as loss of control, defeat, and work-related stress" are associated with obesity and diabetes and a long list of potential side effects. This shows the power of your mind to turn on a host of problems! The good news is, if your mind can turn this stress response *on*...it can also turn it *off*.

To turn off the stress response, we need to:

1. Identify negative self-talk and beliefs.
2. Upgrade your beliefs.
3. Be kind to yourself.

---

[9] Mike Mutzel, *Belly Fat Effect*, 52.

IDENTIFY NEGATIVE SELF-TALK AND BELIEFS

If I were to put a microphone up to your head and we could hear your thoughts, what would they be? Yes, I know there will be crazy things that float through, but over time, what are the regular thoughts that make up the landscape of your mind? How about the ones that have taken up residence and are so comfortable in there you might not even recognize they are there anymore? Those are the thoughts we want to tune into and unpack in this chapter. These thoughts are clues to the beliefs that you hold about yourself. And the beliefs you hold about yourself will determine your experience.

Growing up, I was conditioned to fade into the background. There were other needs and other people more important than me and my needs. This showed up with thoughts like, "I don't matter. My needs don't matter. I'm not that important." No one told me those specific words. At one point in time I had just adopted these beliefs in order to make sense of what was going on around me. As an adult, it would show up when I would say, "I'm fine," even though my husband could tell I was anything but fine. It would show up when I would be giving and giving and giving to the kids all day and end up feeling frustrated and resentful about my situation. I felt like a victim in my own home. When I finally recognized these beliefs and addressed them, I was able to upgrade them. I was able to change them into beliefs that serve me now and help me to feel empowered in my own life.

In *Try Softer*, Aundi Kolber writes, "Many of us have an internal voice that is keeping us stuck, traumatized, unhappy, and alone. This voice reminds us that we are not enough, not worthy, too much, and too little all at the same time. It's not hard to see how this voice impacts our day-to-day lives, is it? If our central narrative is that *we are bad*, then nothing we do will ever be enough—and no amount of behavioral management will fix this wound."[10]

Woah…that's heavy! You might be thinking, "What am I supposed to do with that?!" For now, I am just trying to expose what has already been in your mind. You can't work with it if you don't even know it's there. Just take note of the thoughts you think about yourself. We will work more with these later.

UPGRADE YOUR BELIEFS

In order to change your current experience, you must change your beliefs. As long as I believed that I didn't matter and others were more important than me, I would make choices to confirm that belief. I could not create a new experience for myself until I upgraded my beliefs and made space for a new reality. Until you update these, you will be stuck in your current reality.

If you have a belief, "I will always be this weight" or "I don't deserve more," can you see how that will impact the choices you make and the experience you create for yourself? Can you see this in yourself? What are your common thoughts? What beliefs do you hold about yourself? Do you see how you make choices to confirm these beliefs?

Shad Helmstetter talks about this in *What to Say When You Talk to Yourself*, "When you recognize that we can make a change in our lives by making a change in our programming, you see, for the first time, a crack in the wall of the 148,000 negative doubts and destructive beliefs that each of us has built up in front of us. It becomes clear that what was holding us back, defeating us, can

---

[10] Aundi Kolber, *Try Softer: A Fresh Approach to Move Us Out of Anxiety, Stress, and Survival Mode—and into a Life of connection and Joy* (Tyndale House Publishers, 2020), 193.

itself be defeated, and you realize that an exciting new future is about to become available to anyone who was standing behind the wall, waiting to get through. What an exciting decision to break through that wall!"[11]

Here's the good news—it doesn't have to stay this way! You can do something about this. Are you ready to "break through the wall?" I hope so! Because you absolutely can! Helmstetter continues, "Those of us whose dream it is to improve our lives, even in a small way, can do so. If you want to solve a problem (meet a challenge) or reach any goal, learn to give yourself precise and complete directions. If you have a goal, no matter what it is, wire your brain with detailed instructions that tell you exactly what you want."[12]

In order to achieve your dream for yourself, what detailed instructions do you need to give your brain? These will be your empowering messages that will move you from your current state to your ideal future version of yourself. Remember the vision of your future self from Chapter 4? Maybe you need to remember how confident and satisfied you felt. Maybe you need to remember the smile on your face. To rewire your brain, write out your statements in the "I am…" format. "I am confident." "I am happy." "I know what decisions to make." "I enjoy my family and my job." These statements tell your brain where to focus. They help it know where you are headed and what you are wanting to change, and it will begin working for you to implement these changes. Have you heard the statement, "What you focus on grows"? This is exactly what you are implementing here. What do you want to grow? Do you want your negativity or depressed thoughts to grow? Then,

---

11 Shad Helmstetter, *What to Say When You Talk to Yourself*, 28.
12 Shad Helmstetter, *What to Say When You Talk to Yourself*, 156.

keep focusing on them. Do you want your confidence and self-esteem to grow? Then, focus on positive, affirming, and uplifting statements, activities and thoughts—and they will grow. Don't stay stuck where you are, make the intentional choice to do something different and in time you will become different.

BE KIND TO YOURSELF

Some of you may realize right away that you are not very kind to yourself. Others of you may not even realize how harsh you are to yourself because it has just been your internal landscape for so long. As I mentioned earlier, imagine I am holding a microphone up to your head and we start recording you as you talk to yourself. When you make a mistake, what do you say? When you are going about your daily tasks, what do you say to yourself? What if you spoke out loud every response you say to yourself, but they were directed at your best friend? How would you feel about saying those things to her/him? To begin shifting this, consider Brené Brown's powerful words from *Daring Greatly*:

"[We need]...to give ourselves a break and appreciate the beauty of our cracks or imperfections. To be kinder and gentler with ourselves and each other. To talk to ourselves the same way we'd talk to someone we care about."[13]

I love this: "[What if we] talk to ourselves the same way we'd talk to someone we care about." What if you could do that? Can you feel the difference in what you might say? I know I did when I started implementing this. It was a breath of fresh air to give myself a break and not worry so much and allow myself to be imperfect.

---

13 Brene Brown, *Daring Greatly: How the Courage to Be Vulnerable Transforms the Way We Live, Parent, and Lead* (New York: Avery, 2012), 131.

I could be patient with myself instead of beating myself up for slowing down or letting things go undone. What a burden that has lifted for me! And you know what? My body thanks me for giving it a chance to rest and heal and stay out of the stress state. How about you? What would be different for you if you could implement this? Can you sense a difference in how you would view yourself? How you would feel about yourself?

> ***Take Action:*** What resonated with you most in this chapter? What would you like to journal about? Can you identify your negative self-talk and beliefs? What are they? How would you like to upgrade them? What new beliefs would you like to rewire into your brain? What new "I am" statements resonate with you? Where will you post them to keep them visible? How can you practice being kind to yourself?

Chapter 8
ADJUST YOUR RESPONSES

After reading the last chapter, hopefully you are beginning to notice your thoughts and becoming aware of the positive and negative messages that are common. I hope you are beginning to see how they are impacting you emotionally and physically. In this chapter, we will dive deeper into what is going on in your mind to see if there are any stressors that might be impacting your waistline.

In the last chapter we learned your mind does not discern whether you are experiencing *real* or *perceived* stress. It just receives the message that you are stressed (caused by an external or internal stressor) and sends out the stress signal to the body, which produces more cortisol. As Mike Mutzel explains, this is why we do not want that happening regularly:

"Cortisol sabotages our waistline…first, by preferentially depositing fat in the abdominal region; and second, by stimulating appetite and creating a preference for calorie-rich foods and carbohydrates."[14]

---

14 Mike Mutzel, *Belly Fat Effect*, 53.

This is why I've allocated two chapters of my book to exploring what is going on in your mind—it matters! If you can learn how to be aware of what's going on in your mind and be intentional and proactive with the messages you send to your body, you *will* notice a difference in your waistline.

Think through your day and evaluate stressors that you have to deal with on a regular basis. How stressful is your job? Maybe you are single and worried about if you will find the right partner. Perhaps you are worried every day about your kids and how they are doing academically. Your relationship with your significant other might be strained. Maybe there are family relationships that can cause your chest to tighten and you start feeling overwhelmed and panicky about how to respond to their dysfunctional ways of communicating. I'm stressed just thinking about all of these scenarios! Can you feel that as well?

Or, maybe you are like one of my clients who did not even realize she was stressed. Linda had asked to meet with me to determine why she was stuck in her weight loss journey. She was tracking everything she ate, working out regularly, and cooking very healthy meals. In discussing different areas that could potentially trigger fat storage, I started discussing stress. I asked, "What is your average stress level?" She said, "Not very high." She felt that things were not stressful in her life, things were fine. Further along in our conversation, I mentioned internal stress and how that can encourage the body to shift into fat storage mode. I gave a few examples of what that would look like. She commented, "Well, that's probably my problem! My brain never stops!! I'm constantly worrying about this or that and even though I'm sitting here talking with you I'm worrying about what's next, what's for dinner, wondering if my daughter is doing what she needs to right now…" Bingo! We found it. She did not think she had any stress because she did not feel any from external sources, but internally she lived in a constant state of stress. We compared her brain to a hamster running on his wheel. That's where we focused our coaching time over the next few weeks—uncovering why she stayed in that stressed mental state and began unraveling the web that had contributed to her internal turmoil (I'm happy to report she found freedom—more on that in the next chapter).

Do you resonate with that story? What is your internal landscape? Generally calm? Totally stressed out? Somewhere in between?

Now that you are becoming more aware of your thoughts and your internal stress state, that is huge! You can't fix a problem if you don't know it's there. My hope is that you are beginning to see things you didn't even notice were there before. This is a potential area that can cause you to be stuck in a stressed state and thus turning on the fat storage message in your body. If you knew you could turn off that message, would you want to try? I thought so! The key: *You cannot control what happens to you, but you can absolutely control how you respond.*

Let's start with an external stressor and use the workplace for this example. Imagine you just had a meeting with your boss. She critiqued a report you turned in and told you what she would like to see you do differently next time, then thanked you for your hard work, and the meeting was adjourned. Where do your thoughts go? Do you focus on the one negative comment she made, and start spinning on that one statement and then are unable to think about anything else? Can you see yourself and how this is taking over and consuming your thoughts? Can you feel how this comment is spreading from your head and you are now feeling it all over your body? Your chest might be tightening, your breathing is shallower...and then your mind gets activated. You are going over all the things you have done, how nothing you do is good enough for her, if you were the boss you would run things differently, etc. Can you see how you go from valued worker to just a measly employee in a hot second? Can you feel your body reacting to this? Exactly! You just hit the stress button and sent a wave of stress hormones through your body. Take a deep breath, I know I just did! Breathe...

Let's implement the Adjust Your Responses step and see how you could handle this situation differently...

You are in a meeting with your boss, she shares what she would like you to do differently...you notice your body tensing and you notice all the negative thoughts that are waiting to jump into the scene...you take a deep breath, take a bathroom break, and walk yourself through this. You remember what you like about your boss. You remember the affirming words your boss has said to you before. You remember that you like this job, you like working for your boss. Then, you revisit her comments. You can see the validity of what she said. And then you remember that you did write that report last minute because you were up late with your sick daughter and came in late the morning it was due. So, you take a deep breath, choose to be patient with yourself and your reality—you have a two-year-old daughter and not much family support. You decide to follow up with your boss and apologize, thank her for her patience, and let her know what you will do differently next time.

Can you feel the difference in energy for these two responses? These two options (or variations of them) are your choice. Which one would you rather try? And if you say the first one, remember what is happening internally as you rant and rave...you are putting your body in a state of stress and telling the body to store up for a crisis. For the second response you experience the stress, then find a way to *adjust your response* to take your body out of the stress state, thus turning off the fat storage message.

Now, let's start with an internal stress that can turn into a stressful state of mind. Let's say you look at yourself in the mirror and you think, "Ugh! When am I ever going to lose all this baby weight?" This starts as just a negative thought…you then choose to hold onto that negative thought and go for a ride on that mental roller coaster. "You will never lose this weight. You have no self-control. Your mom is right, you can never complete anything you start. I'm surprised my husband is still with me." And on and on the dialogue continues. Now you are feeling stressed, you have a headache, your stomach is in knots, and you find yourself in the pantry searching for anything to numb the pain.

Phew! Take a deep breath! Does that sound familiar? Maybe the words are a bit different, but can you see the progression? One negative thought can lead to stress, feelings of overwhelm, and your body gets the signal to be prepared for an emergency situation. It slows down metabolism, diverts energy from all non-essential functions, stores energy, and prompts you to eat more high-calorie foods to be ready to react when the crisis comes.

Let's back up the story to the first thought that started it all… "Ugh! When am I ever going to lose all this baby weight?" Pause! Stay in this thought for just a moment. This is where the magic happens. What if you could choose to go down a different path? What if you choose to not get on the mental roller coaster ride? This is when you implement the Adjust Your Responses step. Take a deep breath. Let's go back to Brené Brown's advice from *Daring Greatly*, "[We should] *talk to ourselves the same way we'd talk to someone we care about.*"[15] If your best friend were standing in front of you saying that same thing, what would you say to her? What would the expression on your face be? What would your tone be like? Now, say that same thing to yourself. Literally. Say it out loud. And if you are feeling really brave, stand in front of the mirror and say that to yourself. Can you feel the difference? My guess is you are experiencing that response on a very deep level. This is self-compassion. This is choosing to love yourself and not hate yourself. Do you see the difference that response has on you emotionally and physically? Do you think you could try and practice more of that? Your body will be ever so grateful!

Can you see now why it matters what you think and how you respond to stressful situations? I want you to see that no, you cannot control everything that happens to you, but you *do* have control over how you respond to that stress. You can let it grow and fester and sabotage your weight loss efforts *or* you can learn how to observe the stress, choose how you want to handle it, then adjust your responses for your benefit as well as those around you.

I have a beautiful example of this from a recent coaching time with a client. She shared that she isn't thrilled with her current job. It's a fine job, but it doesn't bring her joy. Due to financial reasons, it is not realistic for her to transition yet. I could hear the disappointment in her tone as she described her current job. Then her whole tone changed as she described the job she would love to have dealing with animals. I could hear the tension she felt—dream job vs. current reality. I challenged her to see it differently. What if her current job is *the very thing* that is building a bridge to the job

---

15   Brene Brown, *Daring Greatly*, 131.

of her dreams? Each day, she is building step-by-step the bridge that will lead to the future fulfilment she craves. She appreciated the new, more positive spin on her current situation and I could almost feel her stress level going down! Now, rather than dreading each day, she can remember the purpose behind her work and know that each day she is one step closer to her dream job.

Take Action: What difference could that make in your life if you implemented this? Think about some of the common stressors in your life—internal and external. Spend some time and imagine how you could walk through these situations differently to minimize the stress signals being activated in your body. This is a great topic to discuss with a safe friend and brainstorm different ways that you can respond to stressful situations. You can even help your friend do the same thing!

Chapter 9

SEEK UNDERSTANDING

This is the chapter I have been waiting to write! I am getting teary-eyed just thinking about you reading this chapter and being in this moment "with" you. I have prayed for the opportunity to share this with you. Please know I am praying for you even now.

At this point in the process, you can feel how we started working with external and surface things and have slowly worked our way down into internal and more emotional things. In the next two chapters, we will be diving deeper. Do you trust me? Are you willing to dig a bit deeper and see what else needs to be *released*?

OUR BODIES HOLD OUR STORY

I want you to know your battle with weight loss is about the weight, but it's not about the weight at all. Clear as mud, right?! Let me try to explain. Your battle is with excess weight, yes, but it also can come from a much deeper place than the excess skin you see externally. So, it's about the weight, but it's not about the weight. Maybe this quote from Aundi Kolber will help:

"The grief, anxiety, fear, or heartache we won't let ourselves feel will come out in other ways… When we don't allow our bodies to process their experiences, they will certainly tell us—even if it means through panic attacks, chronic illness, depression, or more… We know we can try to run from the wisdom and experiences of our bodies; after all, disconnection is one way we make it through uncomfortable relationships and experiences. But the truth is, our memories and experiences do not simply go away. Our bodies are their keepers, for better or worse."[16]

Our bodies hold our story.[17] They can try many ways to get our attention. Aundi mentions "panic attacks, chronic illness, depression, or more." I would like to suggest that included in the "more" could be holding on to excess weight. Consider the excess weight that you are struggling to lose, what untold story might it hold? What unprocessed pain could it be holding?

Remember the client, Linda, I mentioned in the last chapter that was stuck in her weight-loss journey? We worked together for a few months on ways to tame her overactive mind and then landed on a painful memory that she had kept a secret. I challenged her to write a letter to release this memory. After she finished, she sent me a text saying, "I never realized how much 1,437 words really weighed." Wow! That's powerful. I asked how it felt to get that out and see it all in writing. She replied, "Energized, empowered, and relieved." Can you just take a moment and give her a hand clap! That's called bravery. To finally put into words the pain that had been buried for years! She chose to be brave, press

---

16   Aundi Kolber, *Try Softer*, 148.
17   This concept is from Bessel van der Kolk, *The Body Keeps the Score: Brain, Mind, and Body in the Healing of Trauma* (New York: Penguin, 2014).

in and experienced a new sense of freedom that she had never felt before. That is what I'm trying to get you to see—your body could be holding a story that needs to get out.

For me, I had already experienced weight loss, but I know I would have eaten it all back on due to emotional eating if I had not taken steps to secure my freedom. I will share the steps I took to secure my freedom—so that you can secure yours, or find it for the first time!

JOURNALING AND PRAYING

An instrumental book for me has been *A Guide for Listening and Inner Healing Prayer* by Rusty Rustenbach.[18] This taught me how to spend quiet time praying and bringing my pain to God and allowing him to speak into the pain and bring healing to my heart. I have done some counseling, but the most healing that I have experienced has been in my own personal quiet times praying and inviting God into the pain. When you hear God speak love, value and reframe a situation…it's the deepest comfort I have experienced. In *Daring Greatly*, Brené Brown shares a quote from James W. Pennebaker's book, *Writing to Heal*:

"Since the mid-1980s an increasing number of studies have focused on the value of expressive writing as a way to bring about healing. The evidence is mounting that the act of writing about traumatic experience for as little as fifteen to twenty minutes a day for three or four days can produce measurable changes in physical and mental health. Emotional writing can also affect people's sleep habits, work efficiency, and how they connect with others."[19]

---

18 Rusty Rustenbach, *A Guide for Listening and Inner-Healing Prayer: Meeting God in the Broken Places* (Colorado: NavPress: 2011).

19 Brene Brown, *Daring Greatly*, 82.

I had no idea that as I journaled and prayed, I was using "expressive writing" as a tool for healing. I just knew I felt heard, valued, loved and comforted. As I learned to trust God and be more vulnerable and open, He began to reveal more of His purpose for my pain. Not that He willed it or wanted it to happen to me, but how He was using the pain for my good.

PROCESSING MY PAIN

There is a second part to journaling and praying—processing the pain. It's one thing to just write things down, it's another level to put words to your pain and then process it, either by yourself or with someone.

As Brown explains in *Daring Greatly*, "The research team found that the act of not discussing a traumatic event or confiding it to another person could be more damaging than the actual event. Conversely, when people shared their stories and experiences, their physical health improved, their doctor's visits decreased, and they showed significant decreases in their stress hormones."[20]

Woah…not sharing about a traumatic event could be more damaging than the actual event? That's crazy! It's too much for your body to hold all of that. Your body will try to find a way to release some of it, even if you don't cooperate. Whatever pain you have experienced in your life is a part of your story. You can't change that, but you do have a choice in whether you let that pain define you *or* if it becomes a catalyst to make you stronger. It's your choice. I pray you choose to be brave, press in and process your pain and see how God wants to use it to make you stronger.

---

20 Brene Brown, *Daring Greatly*, 82.

There are many ways to process your pain. I have used my journaling and prayer times to process with God while I am in my comfy chair; I process while I'm running; while on my stationary bike; on my yoga mat; I share with my husband; I share with a safe friend. I have also met with counselors to share about my struggles and ask for their advice.

CHANGING THE MESSAGES
The last step is to change the messages you have internalized. A friend introduced me to a ministry called Revelation Wellness® that taught me how to use fitness as a tool to connect with God and process my pain. Working out became a "get to" and something I looked forward to because I not only trained my body, but trained my heart, my mind, and my spirit as well. I went through their group fitness training because I wanted to lead other women in having this same experience. One of the messages they repeat over and over in training is, "Bad news gets stuck in good bodies."[21] We learned how to use fitness as a way to work that bad news *out* of bodies and good news *into* bodies. As lies or negative messages surfaced, I would use my workout times to process these and then release the old messages to allow space for the new, improved messages.

Let me show you how this process works in my life. Here is a sample entry straight out of my journal:

---

21 Revelation Wellness® is a nonprofit ministry that uses fitness as a tool to teach others how to: Love God. Get Healthy. Be Whole. Love Others. https://www.revelationwellness.org

November, 2013

I'm so ticked off right now! I feel betrayed, abandoned, and rejected.

God, what is this stirring up in me? I know that my reaction is stronger to this situation than it should be... When have I felt this before?

I'm remembering a time when I shared my true feelings with dad. I was home, visiting from college. We were standing in the kitchen, I was crying and shared how much it hurts me that he and mom fight so much. How hard it is knowing your parents don't like each other. It was way too much emotion for dad to bear, so he got in his car and left. He didn't get back until later that night and we never talked about it again.

I felt abandoned. Left alone. Feeling the sting of rejection after I shared my heart.

God, where were you when dad left me?

I see you! You are standing in the kitchen with me, holding me as I cried!! Thank you, God, for being with me in that moment.

I'm hearing the phrase, "I will never leave you or forsake you."

I start journaling what I'm feeling and ask God "What is this bringing up for me? What pain point is this highlighting for me?" He might bring up a memory or a word. I identify what I'm feeling in the memory—the pain point. Then, I identify the beliefs I took on from that memory. I then invite God into the memory and ask where he was or what he was doing. He then will answer with an image, a phrase or maybe a scripture that speaks to the situation.[22]

For this specific journal entry, I cried and released the anger and bitterness I felt toward my dad for not being able to handle my emotions. I forgave him for leaving me. Then, I received the comfort and healing God had for me. I thanked him for being with me and loving me, even when my father could not.

Sometimes I will then share this memory and the comfort I received with a close friend. As a way to "seal the healing" and allow it to sink in deeper. Sometimes I may not hear as clearly as this journal entry and I will go for a run or work out and just sit in it and continue to chew on it for a bit. I have been on a run and God has brought a scripture to mind or an answer to the question I journaled about. God doesn't always answer right away…but he *will* answer.

Lastly, it's what will I do with what I have learned? For this journal entry, I realized that I had taken on the belief that "I am alone." When God showed me that He did not leave me and that He was there comforting me, I have a choice. Will I believe and receive the comfort? Or, will I stay in my broken, "Nobody is there for me" belief state? It's my choice. When I chose to release the lie and believe that God is there for me, I am able to walk in the truth that God will never leave me. I can now receive positive messages from God about his love for me, as well as from those around me.

---

[22] If you want to learn more about this process, please read Rusty Rustenbach, *A Guide for Listening and Inner-Healing Prayer*.

As you can see, I took my pain to God, invited him into it, processed the pain, and received deep healing. I don't *have* to reach for food to satisfy deep longings or to numb out. I have found a better strategy than that! God wants the same for you. He would love to speak into your situation, if you will take the time to sit and ask and be still. Will you allow him this opportunity? I promise it will be worth the time and energy you put forth. Not only do I feel whole and healed, but I found my purpose—to help others who are hurting. What could it do for you to practice these steps?

Take Action: Take a deep breath! This chapter went a bit heavier. How are you doing? What is coming up for you? Try to put words to what you are experiencing. What questions do you have? What resonates with you? If you feel ready, you can start journaling some of your experiences.[23] Make sure you have time. As you begin putting words to things, some strong emotions may rise to the surface. Don't be discouraged, it's ok. Give yourself time and space to unpack them. Allow writing to be a safe space to put your thoughts and emotions down on paper. Journaling and going through the process of putting words to your experiences and emotions can bring clarity, freedom and even release. If your emotions start getting too strong (or if you are afraid to start because you think they might be), try reading Aundi Kolber's book *Try Softer*. She teaches techniques like containment and grounding that will help as you process through your pain.

---

23 For a journal prompt sheet, check out www.marjiemetz.com/release-resources

You don't have to go through this alone. Maybe you need to meet with a counselor or reach out to a safe friend and share your heart. If your memories feel too painful or if you experienced trauma that you have not processed yet, I encourage you to seek out a counselor that specializes in trauma healing. They are trained and know how to help you walk through the trauma and understand its impact in your life.

As I processed through my pain, I shared with close, safe friends and regularly reminded myself of truths that comforted me. These truths pulled me out of the past and reminded me of what is true in the present:

- I am not alone, God is with me.
- I didn't know what to do then, but I have support and resources now.
- I may not understand why, but I know God is for me and will use this for my good.

What statements can help you process through your pain?

Chapter 10
ENJOY YOUR LIFE

The title for this chapter may sound simple, but walking it out is far from easy! I know. It took me many years of frustration, anger, hurt, and a lot of unmet expectations to finally realize the power in this simple statement. Let me start with practical reasons why this is important, and then I will move on to personal examples to show the process in my own life.

We have talked about the importance of observing your thoughts and the impact they can have on your body by allowing negative thoughts or circumstances to turn on the stress response. What I want you to see is that if you can turn on the stress response with negative responses, the opposite is true as well…you can release happy hormones and feelings of safety, belonging, and calmness by choosing to focus on positive thoughts and allowing positive emotions. That's why you hear so much emphasis on "count your blessings" and expressing gratitude and writing down those things for which you are thankful. You can literally change what is happening physiologically inside your body with gratitude. That's crazy! By choosing to be grateful and thankful you can be turning off the fat storage messages in your body.

Take Action: Put this to the test! I do an exercise with my clients where I have them imagine a stressful situation that has happened recently and then I ask them to notice and describe what they are feeling in their body. Next, I have them shake it off, practice deep breathing, then imagine a comforting or happy moment in time. I have them notice and describe what they are feeling in their body. Try this on yourself and see what you notice. Can you feel the shift? That's the difference of living in a state of stress and living in a place of gratitude. Once you make the choice of where you will choose to focus your mental and emotional energy, this will determine what you experience in your body and in your day. Try it for a day. I dare you!

For many years, I did not realize how much additional stress I was adding to my situation by dwelling on the negatives and what I wished would happen. I had pushed and strived and literally worn myself out trying to raise four kids, homeschool some of them, and be all that I needed to be for them. I bottomed out. It took about two years for my body to heal and recover. I lost the excess weight, the puffy look, my energy was returning, and I was able to work off my medication. I had been working through my pain and healing emotionally, but there was still a deeper layer God wanted to address. He wanted me to finally be okay being me and learning to be happy in my own life, not wishing for what others had. I wanted to be different from how he had made me. I just couldn't see how I could be enough for the task He had given me. He had to break me down in order to build me up. How do I know that? That's what He told me in my journaling time:

July, 2013

"I can't handle this!"

"I can't do this!"

"I'm done!"

These statements are bubbling up as I remember Jaden as a baby and how he wouldn't stop crying. I remember feeling so done. Feeling like the situation was far beyond what I could handle. How could I not know how to help my own son?! I have had three other children...how could I not know what to do to help him?

Father, that was such a rough time. I know you didn't leave me during that time, even though I didn't feel you there. What truth do you want to communicate to me?

"I have learned the secret of being content in any and every situation, whether well fed or hungry, whether living in plenty or in want.

I can do all this through him who gives me strength." (Philippians 4:12-13 NIV)

During that time, Jesus, where were you?

"Giving you strength."

What were you doing during that hard time?

"For it is God who works in you to will and to act according to his good purpose." (Philippians 2:13 NIV)

Why did it have to be so hard? What did you want to accomplish in me?

"Death of self."

Wow. Ouch. Yes, I can see that. I can see how that hard time taught me dependence on you. There was nothing I could do to make it better. I could only lean into you to help me get through it. That was hard. Thank you for the work that you did in my heart.

What "burden" do I need to surrender to you?

I'm imagining a heavy rock representing all the expectations I put on myself to know what to do, the need to figure it all out and to be able to handle everything. I'm struggling just to try and hold this rock as I lay it at your feet. I hear, "Come to me, all you who are weary and burdened, and I will give you rest. Take my yoke upon you and learn from me, for I am gentle and humble in heart, and you will find rest for your souls." (Matthew 11:28-29 NIV)

Can you hear the pain? The expectations? How I invited God into the pain? The burden I was carrying that I chose to lay down? Here's another example:

November, 2015

Lord, I feel trapped. Trapped in my role as a mother and homemaker. I don't feel qualified. I don't feel capable. I don't feel like I get to exercise my strengths at all. Feels like my current role just highlights all my weaknesses.

Why Lord? Why do I feel so trapped? Why don't I feel free to be me? What do I need?

Father, I don't feel like I do anything well as a mother. I'm not patient enough, kind enough, productive enough, I don't clean the house enough, I don't spend enough one-on-one time with my kids...

I did not hear a response from God that day. Silence did not mean He didn't hear me, He just wasn't ready to reveal the answer...yet.

December, 2015

Thank you, Lord, for the great conversation with Molly last week! It was totally an answer to prayer. We discussed Christian basics, what she is nervous about, the dynamics of our relationship...so many things. For two hours! It was such a healing conversation for us. We cried, we prayed, we committed to having more talk time. Thank you, Lord.

I allowed myself to consider that maybe motherhood is not all about me "doing it all" or being "everything" for my children.

Maybe it's more about *just being available* for them. Can you see the difference that would make in my parenting? In how I viewed myself? And then how that would translate as I related to others?

Phew! Brings tears to my eyes remembering those hard times. Can you see how God was working through them? When I finally learned how to stop striving and release all the expectations, the burdens, the "shoulds"…and rest in who God created me to be…I became the mother my children needed. I was available, safe, and had capacity to be there for them…because I pressed in, dealt with my pain by inviting God into it…then, I was able to truly enjoy the life I had been given.

I had put so much effort and work into my healing journey—physically, mentally, emotionally, and spiritually—that I wanted to do something significant to commemorate all of it. I needed to climb a mountain. My fortieth birthday was approaching, so my awesome husband helped make it happen. We went to Zion National Park with my brother and sister-in-law and hiked to the very top of Angels Landing—described as "strenuous and steep with exposure to long drop-offs."[24] Yes, that is very true! We were having to hold onto chains bolted into the rock so that we didn't drop off the trail…it was perfect! We sat on top for a bit and I just soaked it all in and thanked God for how far he had brought me. The view was beautiful…this had double meaning for me as I could finally look at my life and say the same thing.

---

24 "Angels Landing" taken from https://utah.com/zion-national-park/angels-landing

Take Action: Remember back in Chapter 4 and how I asked you to write out your wish for yourself? Go back and read over it. Sit in it for a moment. Does it still resonate with you? Anything you want to update or revise? Or, anything that seems highlighted to you as you've worked through the questions in these chapters? To enjoy *your* life, is there anything you need to let go? Anything you need to add? What do you want the rest of your story to look like?

For some of you, you may still be having a hard time identifying what it is you want. This might be hard because you tend to be hyper-focused on the needs of others and neglect your own. Naming the needs of those around you would be easier for you. I need you to understand how important this step is. If you cannot identify what it is you want and need…how can you or anyone else meet your needs? You *must* get in touch with your feelings and learn what it is you like and what you want. Your job is to discover *you!*

Chapter 11
YOU ARE WORTH IT!

Congratulations on making it through all of the steps in the RELEASE process! Can you feel the transforming power of these steps if you choose to implement them? My hope is that you will sit in the steps and questions and let them begin to shift the choices you are making and how you are living your life. It's your choice whether this is just another book you read or if it becomes one of your breakthrough moments.

I hope that during this book, you activated your imagination muscle again. I hope that you have expanded the possibilities that you can see for yourself. That's how you start shifting—you *have* to believe that it's possible first, *then* you can start taking action to create that change. I hope you feel excited and activated.

Think back to other books you have read and changes you have wanted to implement. What type of person are you? Do you dive right in and make the changes? Do you sit in them for a bit, hope to change, but eventually get distracted, forget, and stay the same? Or, are you excited, start implementing and then slowly lose interest and eventually stop? Please don't hear judgment in any of those questions! That is not the point I am trying to make—I want you to evaluate your behavior. How do you generally respond to new information—that is what I am trying to help you notice about yourself. Here's why—I want the information in this book to rock your world! I want it to radically change you from the inside out so that those around you say, "Woah, what happened to you?" So, it's important to evaluate your behavior to know what you should do next. You have a number of options, and I will walk you through them.

Option #1: Stay the same. You've read the book, you enjoyed the information, and you can see the value in it, but you really aren't that motivated to implement any changes yet. That's fine if this is you. I appreciate you taking the time to read this book and hope that when you are ready, you will come back to this book and check out the other options. Or, please pass this book on to someone that you think could really benefit from this information.

Option #2: You really identified with a few steps in the process and you can see the value of implementing changes in your life. You have capacity for slow, gradual changes and would like to devote some time and energy to that. If this is you, I would recommend asking a friend to go through this book with you. You can set up a weekly time to connect and discuss the chapter and then ask these questions each week:

- What did I learn from this chapter?
- What seemed highlighted in the chapter? Like it was written just for me.
- What am I going to implement from this chapter? How will I do this?

These are the keys to making real progress—accountability, processing the information with someone who is interested in the material as well, and then taking action.

Option #3: Your heart and mind are so activated right now—you know you must dive *all in* because you do not want to stay where you are another day! Change must happen now! If this is you, you are ready for coaching. Coaching is designed to provide the accountability, support, and stretch that you need to create the transformation you desire in your life. I know because I have experienced that for myself as I have been coached and that's what I am able to create for my clients. If you are interested, I offer a Release Group Coaching program. Check out my website (www.marjiemetz.com) to see my current offerings.

Whatever option you choose, I need you to consider a few obstacles that could get in the way of you making changes. When I work with clients, sometimes just drawing their attention to potential obstacles and eliminating them can make a huge difference in whether they succeed or fail at meeting their goals. I want you to reach *all* of your goals so I am going to set you up for success by helping you to consider some potential obstacles as you implement changes. Would you like that? I thought so!

CHANGE IS HARD

Anytime you try and go against what you have known as normal, there will be resistance. That's why accountability and support are so vital as you try and implement new things. That's why I recommend in Option #2 that you need to meet with a friend that is going through the book with you. If you try to do this on your own... more than likely, it will not happen. That's not because you are not disciplined...it's just human nature to want to stay the same. That's why it feels like you are swimming upstream as you try to implement anything new. You have to spend extra time, energy, and resources to help you implement the changes. That's where a friend comes in to give you the support you need to keep going. On our own, we tend to slip back into what's most comfortable and easy.

LIFE IS BUSY
Our brains can only focus on so much! Life is busy and there are many things trying to grab our attention. If you are serious about making changes, how will you stay focused and on track to make sure that your priorities are happening? It's just too easy to get sucked into the urgency of everyday tasks and lose traction on what really matters to you. This is the benefit of support and accountability...it's a checkpoint to get you in tune with your priorities again. This is why I have a weekly accountability group (to keep me on track personally) and why I sometimes hire a coach (to keep me on track professionally). On my own, I know I will get distracted and off-track in a heartbeat!

EXCITEMENT WILL WANE
I'm sure you have experienced this! You read something, listened to a podcast or watched an inspiring video—you get all excited about what you learned and you are going to transform your life! Within a week, two at the most, you wonder what happened. Where did all of that excitement go? You just don't seem to care as much about changing as you used to. That's because excitement is an emotion and emotions change...quickly. You have to find a deeper

motivation to keep you focused. Remember Chapter 4 and how I had you dreaming and digging deeper and then identifying an anchor? This is exactly why I had you do that. It matters!

> *Take Action:* Now it's time to make a choice: Look back over Options #1, #2, and #3. Where are you? Are you content to stay the same? Are you wanting to make a few changes? Or, are you desperate to create something new in your life? What will you do about this? If you choose Option #2, who will you ask to go through this book with you? How often will you meet/talk with them? If you choose Option #3, decide how much time, energy, and resources you have available to devote to your transformation.

Before I wrap up this chapter, please revisit your wish from Chapter 4. Sit in that for a moment. Imagine that version of yourself. How much would it be worth to you to have this dream for yourself fulfilled? What would that mean to you? That's what you have to hold onto as you evaluate what you want to do moving forward. Your choices matter. Each day. They can add up to a fulfillment of the dream, or they can keep you in your current situation—feeling stuck, limited and frustrated. Imagine what could be possible for you if this dream were fulfilled. Imagine the new choices that are available to you from this place. Imagine the impact on your confidence, how you view yourself, the impact on your family, your friends. What do you want that to be? And are you willing to purposefully cause that to happen? That's the real question. What are you willing to *do* to create this for yourself and your family? I promise you, it will be worth it! You will not regret the time you invest in your personal growth—*everyone* wins when you make the brave choice that you are worth it!

Chapter 12
WHAT DO YOU WANT?

I remember writing in my journal, "God, please, can I start a new chapter in my story? I am so sick and tired of being stuck in this chapter! Going around and around the same issues, I can't take it anymore!" That cry for help preceded another breakthrough for me. After that, I learned that I didn't have to be a victim of my circumstances anymore. I could make choices to either confirm the old beliefs I had about myself or I could create new ones. I held the power of choice in *my* hands—would I use it and be proactive? Or, would I continue waiting for someone to rescue me? I thanked God for the timely information and got busy creating something new in my life. I made choices that I'm proud of—I hired a coach; I started a group coaching program; I started writing this book; I stepped out in faith to do what I feel called to do. I chose to break free from what I had known. I knew there had to be a better way and God illuminated the path for me to find it. For me the saying has been absolutely true, "A breakdown happens right before a breakthrough."

That is exactly what I want for you. All the pain, the frustration, the stuck-ness, I want you to see it all through the lens of opportunity! An opportunity to grow, learn, and invite God in and ask for perspective. Life can be hard, yes, but it's your choice whether you are miserable through it or let the pain strengthen you. Some of your pain may come from years of being on this weight loss journey. Try to consider, what is the gift in that? How has that served and helped you? Has it increased your compassion for others? Have you grown in wisdom with what works and what doesn't? Have you developed perseverance? How has that grown you as an individual? What do you have to offer others as a result of your struggle? My hope is that you will press in, find the messages your story holds for you, and transform your pain into your purpose. What could it look like for you to commit to your growth? To press in, dig deep, and uncover the hidden messages in your body's story?

I know you picked up this book because you have been stuck in your weight loss journey. I hope that now you can see there are many layers to why your body can be stuck. I hope and pray that as you continue on your journey that you will receive all that you desire. I also want you to know that your value and worth are not tied to the number on the scale. There is so much more to what determines the measure of your health and value than just that number. Working on weight loss is fine, just don't let it consume you and don't believe the lie that one number determines your worth. You are way more complex and valuable than that! God has specifically designed you with gifts and talents unique to you. Your family, friends, and the world benefit from you walking in your divine design. You make the world a better place as you learn to walk in your gifts and talents. Don't be selfish! Cultivate and grow those gifts.

I hope you have felt my love and concern for you through these pages. This has definitely been a labor of love for me and it's my desire that it has touched you in some way. If I had to boil my message down to one statement, it would be this: *healing, whether physically, mentally, emotionally, or spiritually, only comes when we press into the pain and not avoid it.* As you saw in my breakthroughs, I found the answers, the healing, and the freedom by pressing into the pain. You can too.

I will end with this: I want you to imagine yourself confident; happy; fulfilled; physically, mentally, emotionally, and spiritually healthy; at peace, strong and a champion for yourself and your family. What changes do you need to make for that to be true for you? Whatever they are—*go do them*! You get one shot at this life, make the most of it and don't hold back. You don't want to get to the end of your life and think, "If only...." Don't do that to yourself! Take action and go after what you want! You have been put on this planet, at this point in time…for a specific purpose, go accomplish it!

ACKNOWLEDGEMENTS

This book would not have been possible without the love and support of my husband and my kids. Eric, thank you for encouraging me to keep pressing in and for managing the kids, being understanding of our messy house, making dinner so I could keep writing, and for believing in me even when I didn't believe in myself. John, James, Molly, and Jaden, thank you for being understanding while I focused on the book more and on my role of mom less. Thank you for stepping up and managing things on your own so that I could focus; for listening to me process and share frustrations; and for giving me high fives when there was a milestone to celebrate. I love that we get to do life together.

Thank you to my accountability group—Gail, Jen, and Marnie—for holding a safe space for me during our weekly meetings. Your friendship, love, support, and prayers kept me going so many times when I wanted to just give up. I am blessed to have you in my life.

My Revelation Wellness® fitness ladies are the best! Not only do we workout together, we have also supported each other through many ups and downs over the years. Thank you for your big hearts and for supporting me on this journey. It is a joy and an honor to lead class for you all!

I love my clients (you know who you are)! Thank you for trusting me, for sharing your story, and allowing me the honor of walking part of your journey with you. What a joy it is to see you come alive and walk in freedom!

To my other family members, my friends, mentors, doctors, and practitioners who have supported me on my journey, thank you. I know I would not be where I am today without your help and support.

I would also like to thank God, my Heavenly Father, for all the love, encouragement and gentle, but persistent prodding to encourage me to write. The first time I sensed the whisper, "Write down your story," I thought it was crazy talk! Who am I? I am not a writer! But, thank you, God, for seeing in me what I couldn't see. You put a story inside of me and your love and persistent grace gave me the strength to let it out. Thank you.

ABOUT THE AUTHOR

MARJIE METZ

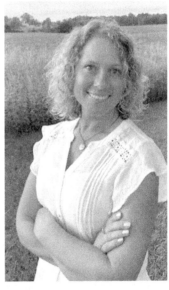

Marjie graduated from Bluffton University with a Food and Nutrition: Dietetics degree. After graduating, she married her college sweetheart, started a family and chose to focus on raising their four, active and fun kiddos for many years. After struggling with mild depression/anxiety, brain fog, weight gain and low energy, she learned how to support and work with her body to overcome these issues. She became a DIET FREE® Facilitator, as well as a certified Health and Life Coach through the Health Coach Institute® to help women struggling with these issues through group and one-on-one coaching programs.

Marjie also learned that health is more than physical in nature and had to work through deep emotional wounds to gain emotional and spiritual healing. Through journaling and faith-based workouts, she found freedom. She wanted to share that with others, so she became a certified Revelation Wellness Fitness Instructor® to help women work out the negative messages and beliefs that keep them stuck.

Marjie is passionate about coaching, speaking and teaching fitness classes to inspire women to lose what weighs them down so they can have energy, love their life and be who God created them to be.

Marjie and her husband, Eric, have been married for 20 years; live near Cincinnati, Ohio; and enjoy the journey with their four amazing children—John, James, Molly and Jaden.

What's next?

Scan the QR code below to gain access to my exclusive video and resources to help you continue on your journey!

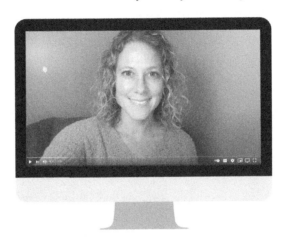

Bonus resources:

Video teaching on: "What's Next?"

RELEASE Summary Page

www.marjiemetz.com/release-book

Let's Stay Connected!

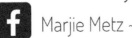 Marjie Metz ~ Health & Life Coach

 @metz4health

Testimonials for:

RELEASE GROUP COACHING PROGRAM

"The group provided a support group that together we came up with great ideas and creatively problem solved, all while Marjie asked furthering questions, pushing us to analyze ourselves. I feel like **my quest for personal discovery is insatiable** now that I've made this great big leap! I'll continue to train myself on positive talk, fellowship without food, and eating with purpose."
—S. Lawrence

"This group program helped me have more baby steps defined, **more hope and a vision for overcoming.**"
—Michelle D.

"My homework of looking into the mirror and what I saw at the beginning and end of this program shows how much I changed. At the beginning of the program, I saw an ugly, lazy, puffy, in pain, having heartburn, unhappy with self, unorganized, unsure of what to do, hiding behind clothes, uncomfortable and stuck in bad habits person. By the end of the program, I saw a new mindset: my self-put-downs became possibilities and I was intrigued and hopeful! I learned that one of my biggest problems was how critical and mean to myself I was. I began learning how to be kind to myself; to see struggles as a chance to work through issues with the Lord; **having joy in the struggle.** I learned that being mean to myself when I was stuck accomplished nothing, but **being kind to myself and looking for the real need under the behavior,** helped me see what the real issue was. Then I could change things and move forward. Many times, it was not about food. When the mental blocks were identified and removed, **losing weight became much easier and enjoyable.** Instead of fighting against myself, I learned to work with myself.

—LM

Made in the USA
Columbia, SC
25 September 2023